I0435488

For the Father God and His Son Jesus Christ, who motivated me to encourage others in pursuit of good health

TABLE OF CONTENTS

INTRODUCTION

The goal is to encourage the pursuit of good health starting now and understand how to achieve it. Good health *can* be achieved and maintained throughout life without breaking the bank or the "head bone". The fact is people have the right to know what is available in the category of health and health care. They have a right to choose the direction to go and the right to maintain what is best for them.

Contained in these chapters are brief insights and encouragement about healing the digestive system to boost immunity; fight cancer; lose weight; recover from irritable bowel syndrome; balance hormones and increase libido; reverse allergies, autoimmunity and osteoporosis with foods and herbal remedies. Everything in the body is connected and affects every other part so looking at the whole and how it works is good idea.

Then it will take time to digest what is said here (no pun intended), take time to research the particulars of your goals to good health, and then apply it in everyday life. Be convinced that this *truly is* a need not only for *you* to function and feel good but because others around you rely on you, are influenced by you, and *need you*. In order to get anything done in life, a mindset of learning and persistence will enable you to "Live a Lifetime of Good Health" in service to God and humanity.

Chapter 1 – What is your motivation? Who, when, why, how?

The American athlete and baby boomer Jim Ryun said, "Motivation is what gets you started. Habit is what keeps you going." I might add, what comes between them is what happens between your ears – thoughts and where they lead you.

What motivates you? What habits will you form? Your motivation and the habits you form will guide you to the kind of successful and long-lasting health you want to achieve.

What is the thought behind the habit? Successful habits come as a result of thought and repetition so make sure that you put enough brain and will-power into changing what you do. Base it on what you learn. When you understand why, it's a lot easier to build the right habits.

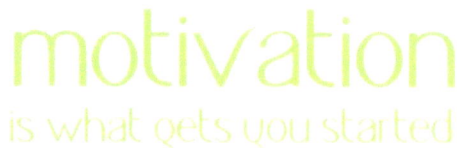

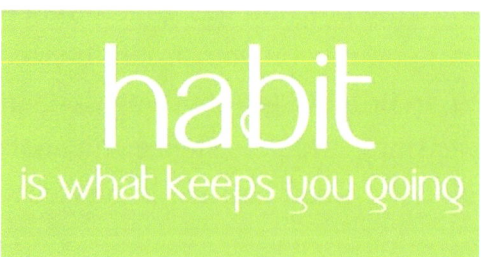

You probably don't need me to tell you how important good health is to you now and in the future. Most people agree that good clean food and some regular activity or exercise is good for them but few take time to figure out what that means to *them*. It may seem simple to *decide* to do something but seem impossible to start. Believe me; I know how it feels to have so much information its overwhelming. But there's hope because decision is a great start so you're already on your way!

I'm Christian and a reader and a believer of Biblical principle, so I know God wants me to be healthy. Other Christians may *want* to know and dearly *need* to know how to achieve it, but non-Christians can benefit from better health as well. Credit where it's due, remembering the One Who gave us these bodies and knowing all about how it works, the Heavenly Father God said what He meant and meant what He said here:

3 John 2 (KJV)

Beloved, I wish above all things that thou mayest prosper and be in health, even as thy soul prospereth.

I know life is busy. As a Biblical research, teaching, and fellowship student for over 40 years and practicing commercial interior designer for over 30 years, these activities took much of my time. After the last project before retirement, I decided to focus on my next passion: improving and maintaining good health which also encompasses another great interest – organic gardening.

Part of *my* motivation is to help other people find direction and clarification in the subject of health so they can get motivated about *their* health. What I did might help others have better health, too. No one arrives at their destination without planning and I'm a lot closer than I was over 10 years ago. Although it may not be exactly the same direction you decide to pursue, it might strike a chord if I may use a musical term, (something else of interest to me).

I digress a little but the point is that no matter how busy you are or how many interests you have, it takes focus and determination to divert some of your energy *now* so you'll have the energy *later* to do whatever you love to do when you grow older and retire…so why wait?! Why not start now?!

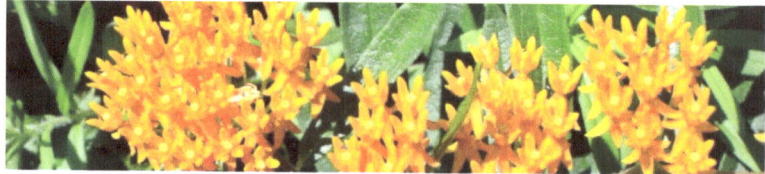

One of the things "boomers" are known for is not letting age keep us from doing the things we love. Not much can stop us except our health, if we let it. We know if we cut ourselves, we can put a band aid on it to keep it from getting dirty, but even without a band aid, it still heals. That's how our bodies are made – to heal. The various body systems work together in a very connected way and there are foods we can eat; things we can do to maximize immunity and healing for the body.

Food is medicine. You don't need a doctorate or even a certificate in nutrition, although it helps to find out more about nutrition and your body. You don't need prescription drugs, except in dire situations until health can be restored.

All that's needed is good organic food and pure filtered water for your life and healthy activities to bring natural solutions for a lifetime. Your body will reward you with vitality and immunity from any disease the world can throw at you. Just like managing any project, in this case *you*, it's work but it's very worthwhile, too.

That said, I urge you to find your own health priority and work on that issue first. My priority was the digestive system. I dare say, if you have *any* physical challenges, most will also find this at the bottom of their issue, no pun intended. So if you don't know why you're feeling tired, run down, without energy, or getting sick all the time, I suggest you start with the gut.

Hippocrates, the father of modern medicine, was a wise man. Much of his wisdom, which is now over 2000 years old, has stood the test of time.

"ALL DISEASE BEGINS IN THE GUT." – Hippocrates

Anyway, the digestive tract was the first thing I attacked. I mean "attacked" in a figurative sense, of course, because there's so much information on the web that I really needed to stay focused on the real issues and believe I would find exactly what I needed to know on my quest for good health. As a result of that belief, I was able to find exactly what I needed quickly because God was at work in my life:

Philippians 2:13 (NIV)

"For it is God who works in you to will and to act in order to fulfill his good purpose."

Another challenge I considered was the beliefs held by different generations about good health and the different ways they go about achieving it (or missing it). My mother worked in a hospital where one of her jobs was making sure the surgical tools in the operation room were sterile. Her view of medicine tends to be conventional and runs the gamut from vaccinations to antibiotics and pain pills (in fairness, she's 83 now and in chronic pain so medication makes it bearable).

My mother's generation generally believed that if what they ate was good enough for their parents, it was good enough for them. For the most part, food was of better quality than food available to us now because it has degraded and been poisoned – chemicals are used for fertilization; herbicides keep to off the bugs, hormones and vaccinations to supposedly make them bigger and disease resistant.

The other spectrum is the generation after my own, the Millennials are aware of the dangers of GMO's' (Genetically Modified Organisms), air and water pollution, unrenewable resources and other environmental issues. They prefer to eat organic non-GMO food that hasn't been treated with hormones, chemical fertilizers, and pesticides.

Of course, I stand in the middle, a baby-boomer, and living the best of both worlds: Conventional medicine tests for disease in the body and prescribes something to subdue the symptoms momentarily. Functional Medicine addresses the source, guiding the body to the proper balance, to heal itself 'whole-istically' the way it was designed by God.

Most of my generation, (the 60-somethings), still muddle through both sides of these worlds at times, and are dying of degenerative diseases, such as cancer, heart disease, ALS, etc., at an increasingly alarming rate. Degenerative disease has been defined as "the result of a continuous process based on degenerative cell changes, affecting tissues or organs, which will increasingly deteriorate over time, whether due to normal bodily wear or lifestyle choices such as exercise or eating habits." What habits will offset degenerative disease then? We need to return to the ways God set up for our health. It's time for our generation to change direction and everyone else will benefit from our example.

This isn't the first time baby-boomers blazed a trail out of necessity (taken from Wikipedia 12-22-15):

> **1945-1947 - World War II** veterans return home from Europe and the Pacific in droves. The wounded had begun returning earlier.

> **July 27, 1953 - Korean War** ends and veterans return home.

May 17, 1954 - U.S. Supreme Court desegregates schools in Brown v. Board of Education. Boomers are the first elementary school generation to attend integrated schools.

June 23, 1960 - The FDA approves an oral contraceptive, Enovid (The Pill), for sale in the U.S.

1964-1975 - Vietnam War, the war boomers fought in and protested against. The average age of combat soldiers is 19.

Summer 1967 - The "Summer of Love", the **hippie counterculture** of sex, drugs and rock n roll.

1968 - Women's Liberation and the feminist movement begins. The oldest boomers are 22.

August 15-18, 1969 - Woodstock, a music festival in Bethel, New York takes place, where more than 400,000 people attended and more than 30 acts perform.

December 1, 1969 - The **first Selective Service lottery since 1942** is held. The lottery is for armed forces inductees for 1970. Only males 18-26 are eligible. September 14 is drawn first. The oldest the boomers are 23.

January 22, 1973 - Roe vs Wade makes **abortion legal** in the United States.

March 12, 1975 - The **last Selective Service lottery**. The oldest boomers are 29. The system is suspended on April 1 and registration for the draft is suspended in January 1976.

1979 - The year the U.S. **divorce rate peaks**. There are 2,331,000 marriages and 1,181,000 divorces, according to the U.S. Census, and the first of the boomers turn 33.

July 1980 - Selective Service registration is **revived** for all males born 1960 and later. The youngest of the boomers will be 16 by year's end.

March 9, 1983 - Legislation passes **raising the retirement age**, with full Social Security benefits, from 65 to 67 to begin in 2000.

January 20, 1993 - Bill Clinton (August 19, 1946), is sworn in as the 42nd president of the United States, the **first boomer in the White House.**

January 1, 1996 - The **first of the baby boomers turn 50**.

January 1, 2011 - The first of the **boomers turns 65**. Approximately two-thirds of all seniors 65 and over and 60% of those 50-64 have at least one chronic disease.

June 25, 2015 - Millennials outnumber baby boomers with 83.1 million people in the U.S. born between 1982 and 2000.

Our heads spin with the volumes of research, technology, and information obtained and utilized for the world's benefit. Why not take advantage of that knowledge for our personal health? It finally hit me when I was prescribed a drug the doctor said I would have to take for the rest of my life! I had to admit I wasn't in good health. I couldn't have children.

Antibiotics didn't work on me anymore. I developed an ulcer from taking ibuprofen on an empty stomach. I had chronic pain in my abdomen identified as irritable bowel syndrome. I eventually had surgery to remove an obstacle (probably scar tissue) in my stomach from the ulcer. I felt awful and had no energy. Something had to change – that something, that *someone* was me! After all, *I am the only person I can change.*

Even though there are steps we can take to improve our health, few find the energy to do more than they're already doing in this busy world. Families with kids run them to and fro for different activities, get them to school, get off to work and home again so you can fix a meal to fill their stomachs.

What happened to you in this equation? Life and food are much more meaningful than this rush and flush of commotion just so there's food enough to fill the void in your stomach. Set your priorities; Consider quality and quantity; Establish meaningful spiritual and physical objectives; and don't budge from them or you might wonder what happened to you someday!

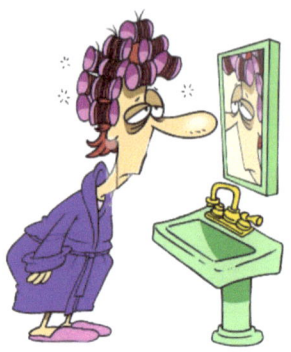

Remember I said the only person you can change is yourself? You can change if you want to change. Never let anyone tell you it's too difficult to do! It's not too late to start! You can do it! And if I can make changes at an advanced age of 54 and into the current age of 64, then it's possible – you can do it, too!

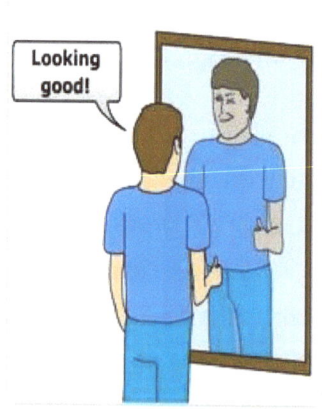

I approach health as a Christian interested in better health personally. It's based on the truth that life is spiritual, there's *nothing I can't do* because it's God in Christ in me, God is good always, and it's not too late to take care of the body God gave me. He designed it to HEAL even if I wasn't a professed Christian.

Suggestion: Start with "The Truth About Cancer: A Global Quest" (TTAC) to get good solid evidence-based reasoning behind what inspired me and listen for your particular health need. It's not just about cancer but general good health practices.

http://thetruthaboutcancer.com/ &

http://www.cancertruth.net/ "The Truth about Cancer" (5 min. Trailer)

http://thetruthaboutcancer.com/video-how-do-you-get-cancer/ (6:40 minute explanation) "Cancer does NOT have to be a death sentence."

https://go.thetruthaboutcancer.com/?a_aid=1589396&a_bid =87aca0ed

There are many books that cite research, one of which is Ty Bolinger's book called *"CANCER: Step Outside the Box"*. It's great for referencing or reading segments of interest without reading the entire volume. That's why I don't get into reference material here, but once you get started on this fascinating subject, you might want to know more. Well, honestly, not everyone will be glued to the subject, but I assure you if you do apply practices of good health, eating right, being active, you'll be rewarded with good health.

Don't we all want to *live a lifetime of good health? It's possible!!*

Chapter 2 – What is Your priority? Where to start?

When I started this quest 10 years ago, I really needed a clear path but it didn't open up to me until I took the first step: I decided something needed to change in my life physically. I ignored my body's needs for years until it couldn't respond as a healthy body should respond. Therefore, since it took years to get into this predicament, it's unreasonable to expect to undo the damage overnight. But happily, since I've started to do something about it, I'm healing quicker and feeling better than I ever dreamed possible!

Decide what you want to achieve and list them under "Goals" at the end of this chapter. Also provided are pages for notes or thoughts as you read. Writing them down helps keep them in front of you and reminds you to stay on track.

If I can do it, you can do it.

Ephesians 3:20 KJV

"Now unto him that is able to do exceeding abundantly above all that we ask or think, according to the power that worketh in us,"

Wow, so is that all?! YES – the first thing you need to do is DECIDE you're going to take positive measures to change, whether it's spiritually, mentally, physically, or emotionally – whether you are sick of being tired or tired of being sick – whatever the problem, you first decide to take it on because if you don't, who will?

If I can do it, you can do it.

Also, perfect practice yields perfect results. Well, perfection is in the Lord, so don't be too hard on yourself or expect it will clear up in a day, a week, a month, or even a year, although there should be improvement in a very short time. Patience and diligence is required but miracles do happen – you'll be rewarded. Let God work in you!

If I can do it, you can do it. Decide you can do it!

Philippians 2:13 KJV

"For it is God which worketh in you both to will and to do of his good pleasure."

Decide you want to Live A Lifetime of Good Health!! Good health is what God wants for us (3 John 2) so it's possible to be healthier than you ever were in your life, no matter what it LOOKS like right now. If you ignore your body, it won't be ready to fend off disease and ailments this fast-paced culture produces.

Even if you're not a follower of God or the Lord Jesus Christ, the body was made to respond to the right treatment and care. The grace of God today, not consequences of the past, dictate an improvement in how you feel and in how well you function if you give your body the nutrition it needs, no matter how badly it was treated in the past. The past is past. It doesn't exist. Learn from it then let it go. Press toward the high calling of the new you.

If I can do it, you can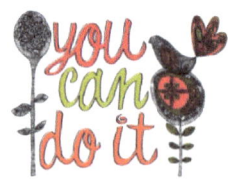

Write Down Your Goals:

1)

2)

3)

Live.Life.Healthy

Chapter 3 – What caused the problem? Get to the bottom of it...

Now that we've established that your body is designed to heal itself, we're supposed to be healthy, so it's time to get to the source of the problem. Ask yourself, "Why am I tired and lack energy? Why am I on this medication? Does it treat the cause or just the symptoms?" If you're unhealthy, your body can't deal with dis-ease the way it was designed to ease-ily take care of whatever came along. You need to get to the source of the dis-ease and restore immunity and health. Yes, it's possible to live a better quality of life.

Find out what the "dis-ease" in your body is. The immune system in our bodies is made to take care of anything that comes our way because we've been fully equipped to handle it. But if you're sick, something's not right. The balance that's off right now just needs to be restored.

Prayer or meditation is essential in this equation. It is a believing effort and as such it is an action verb. It's a thankful state of mind and results in peace of mind. Then we need to get up and do something to build back that part that is lacking or at least do the best you can. That action is an act of positive believing that shows *you can do it*.

2 Timothy 3:17 KJV

"That the man of God may be perfect, thoroughly furnished [equipped] unto all good works."

No matter what arguments your mind is screaming, it's a lie if it contradicts what is available in God's plan. It's possible to be in good health as our soul (mind) prospers. (3 John 2) Remind yourself often of this because there are plenty of times someone will say something contrary and you need to be ready to call the foul (like the referees do in sports), and get back on track. Make it your business to get to know God's will if you are in doubt and want to know. This will go a long way in getting or staying healthy if you aren't already convinced you can do it. The mind is a powerful tool so use it to your advantage.

Prepare your mind every morning to stay on top of your goals. Tell yourself, "No matter what happens today, God already knew it would happen and has taken steps to handle it". Just relax and trust Him. If you're saying, "Easier said than done", I understand. I've had the benefit of getting to know God for over 40 years and every day is "…the day the Lord has made. I will rejoice and be glad in it." (Psalm 118:24) It gets easier the more you trust in the way He has put life into motion.

That said, it's not required that you be a Christian to be healthy. There are plenty of examples of positive believing people to prove it and plenty of self-help books on positive thinking. The human body is a marvelous thing and responds to real food, moderate activity, and healthy positive thoughts, no matter where you're at spiritually. There are no limits put on the human race, so great is the time, the grace, in which we live!

You are what you believe and you can do it if you believe you can do it!

Now, I'm not saying we can live forever if we treat our bodies right but we can live longer, happier, and healthier than we might think is possible. Part of it has to do with what we eat and part of it is the thoughts we allow to lodge in our brains – what we think or dwell on affects our health. If you're fearful of some dreadful thing or another happening, there will be an actual negative chemical effect on your body. If we confidently take on life with a positive attitude, grateful for life, you will be amazed with the positive effect it has on your health!

Notes:

Chapter 4 – What is available? You won't know if you don't ask...

What is the standard for good health? The standard is based on what God made available when we were born, providing everything we need to do it. He gave us food: vegetables, nuts, berries, and herbs when we needed specialized healing. Later, mankind started to eat meat.

Ask yourself why medical doctors prescribe pills and/or surgery for ailments? Well, they're not being taught what it takes to promote healing God's way. All they're taught is to prescribe drugs – they're not taught nutritional healing. That's why we hear more and more about the search for cures for cancer, diabetes, MS, ALS, and all the other degenerative dis-eases. Drugs are merely a stop gap measure that masks symptoms, they are not a cure. You will never hear of a cure until they stop trying to use drugs to do it.

In the previous chapters, I make reference to TTAC (The Truth About Cancer) and once you hear this series, my work is done. What I am striving to do is encourage you because even though it might seem intimidating right now, you need to find out what is available so you can do something about your particular situation. Some key phrases to look up are: gut health, Institute of Functional Medicine, The Truth about Cancer, and clean organic food. Simply put, get started learning more about health issues from people who are concerned about getting to the source of the problem and your symptoms will improve or go away completely!

Look into pertinent subjects about your issue(s), ask questions, assess how it applies to you, and basically find out what will put your body back into balance. It will be different for you than for me. For example, I had surgery to remove scar tissue caused by taking a drug on an empty stomach. It caused other problems, too, such as "dumping syndrome" because that part of my pylori that kept food in my stomach until ready to go to the small intestine was removed. So I eat less at a time and I sometimes lie down for 20 minutes until it can process food I just ate.

What you learn is best for you now might change over time, but you will develop a habit and it's easier to modify it once you set up a routine. The neat thing about life is that you never stop learning so don't be too concerned just because you don't know where this will lead. It's an adventure worth taking!

Something that you can do right away is to eat organic, non-GMO food. Shun processed food. The body handles gradual change better so if you can't eat 100% organically now, work up to it. Check labels. The less ingredients, the better – and avoid eating anything you can't pronounce. Even if you don't have a store that sells organic food near you, find a local organic farm that delivers to a central location. Try Thrive Market *https://thrivemarket.com*

Eating less (especially when you're older) is much healthier. Proportions are important: no more than 1/3 (3-4oz.) of your plate should be meat and at least 2/3 of it should be colorful vegetables.

Every meal does not need to contain meat. We eat far too much meat in the United States for our own good. Eat organic and grass-fed meat as much as possible.

Check out the lacto-fermentation process and make foods like kimchi or sour pickles at home because they contain probiotics that help the digestion and absorption of nutrients.

Another thing to consider is that early mankind didn't sit down to a plate full of food. They didn't always have meat available. They ate what was available like fruit, nuts, or berries they found throughout their active day. They were taught the benefits of herbs passed down through the generations.

Certain diets like "Eat Right for Your Blood Type" or meal plans catering to your particular needs already mentioned in this book help assure proper nutrition.

Acquire a nutritional medicine reference book or two. Find and save websites that aid in gathering information like one called, *http://saveourbones.com/*.

Be a "health nut" and learn what works for you. I will be forever indebted to the first one who told me, "Do your research". I did and I still have my gall bladder with prayer and using herbs and spices.

Right here it needs to be said that if you think organic food and pure water is more expensive, you'd be right. However, it isn't a lot more money for the quality in clean nutrition and in taste. Keep in mind that most people eat too much food, therefore if they ate less, they wouldn't need to buy as much food and if they slow down as well, they will enjoy it even more!

I'm accustomed to budgeting for things so maybe you're already thinking about doing without things you don't really need. But consider this as well: If you're healthier, you wouldn't need to visit the doctor as much (time, gas, wear and tear on you and your car) and forfeiting money for co-pays or prescriptions! That's value added!

Genesis 1:29-31a KJV

"And God said, Behold, I have given you every herb bearing seed, which is upon the face of all the earth, and every tree, in the which is the fruit of a tree yielding seed; to you it shall be for meat [food].

And to every beast of the earth, and to every fowl of the air, and to everything that creepeth upon the earth, wherein there is life, I have given every green herb for meat [food]: and it was so.

And God saw everything that he had made, and, behold, it was very good."

Oh by the way, early civilizations didn't require pesticides, insecticides, or hormones so they would be bigger, therefore considered better – probably wouldn't have even occurred to them. They probably enjoyed eating clean food, real food, just the way it came from nature and therefore ate healthy food. What a concept!

Notes:

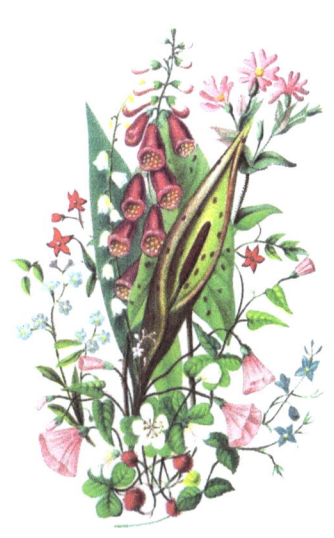

Chapter 5 – What else do I need to know? Unexpected options...

Prepare to be surprised and amazed at what you will find out in this age of information. It can be downright exciting but some of it might not be what you need to know right now. If you find yourself getting sidetracked by the sea of healthful options, step back and remember your particular needs (goals) and focus on them.

What I found out ultimately is that most everything gets down to the health of your digestive system. If you think about it, that's how your body processes and distributes the nutrients in food so if that system isn't working properly, your body won't get the nutrition for the other systems of the body to function.

Good gut bacteria needs to be at least 80% over bad bacteria. Probiotics help take up where roughage leaves off, providing additional good bacteria for digestion and assimilation. Body PH is important to maintain slight alkalinity – disease occurs in acidic conditions.

Disease feeds on sugar so that's why it's vital to cut down on it or better yet, do without or use healthier natural options like honey or stevia. Less is more, put in design terms. The less sugar, the better off you are in the long run.

Sometimes out of necessity, we can add organic nutritional food-based supplements, digestive enzymes, and probiotics to our regimen that help digest and facilitate digestion if you aren't getting the proper amounts of meat, vegetables, and fiber in your diet.

Food supplements take up the slack until you learn what you should be eating to provide your body with the components it needs for good health.

Basically everyone needs a certain amount of water, vitamins, minerals, and roughage for elimination to thrive. Artificial chemical-based supplements can't be utilized in your body – the natural body needs natural or real food sources. This eliminates processed food, food in a box, fast food, which is what most people on a fast-paced lifestyle live on. No wonder there's so much ill health going on!

And I haven't even said much about water – do I need to go into it? I think most people know they need to drink it but are confused about how much water to drink. Here's where you need to think about how much liquid you drink and how active you are. Logically, if you don't consume much liquid and/or have an active lifestyle, you need more water. If your lips are chapped, drink water. Common sense is useful here – it's a balance.

Food is at its highest level of nutrition and most beneficial when it's organic and raw so that's another concept to wrap your mind around. RAW? Yes, I'm not 100% there yet either! I do eat more raw food than in the past and actually have acquired a taste and even a desire for them. Organic food is much tastier and has more flavor than processed food anyway. So why not eat better tasting food?! I found a great casserole using raw (puree of) sweet potatoes that was absolutely delicious – served it at Thanksgiving and no one was the wiser!

When you do cook, use low heat for a prolonged period, like a crockpot on low, so the nutrition will be retained in the broth. High heat destroys nutrients – raw is better as a goal. Juicing or smoothies are beneficial.

As the food provider for your loved ones, ask yourself what you want to give them to eat. Better yet, ask yourself what you want to eat and drink – everyone benefits!

You might consider consulting professionals who can help you along the way. Some of the things you hear about or read will "make sense" to you. You'll just know it's what you need to hear. Just start with what you know and live one day at a time.

Learn about functional medicine. Here's a website to help find a functional medicine doctor in your area but talk to them about their specialties:

www.functionalmedicine.org\practitioner_search.aspx

And remember, *if I can do it, you can do it.*

A little help doesn't hurt, either.

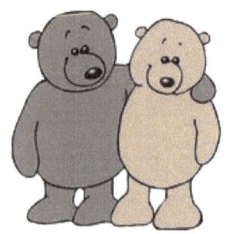

Chapter 6 – How do I know it's working? Tracking results...

I highly recommend when you start out that you find document templates something like the ones you see below to track your progress. You might like a Microsoft electronic version you can use on your computer. There are mobile applications like "MyFitness" that are designed to track various parts of your progress and are fairly user friendly.

Make note of the process: Was it difficult, take too much time, or have an adverse reaction? Alter or edit these examples according to your use. Have fun with it!

Meal Schedule

[Name]

Week # 1	4-Jan-16 – to – 10-Jan-16				
Day	Morning	Afternoon	Notes	Evening
Monday				
Tuesday				
Wednesday				
Thursday				
Friday				
Saturday				
Sunday				
Week # 2	11-Jan-16 - to - 17-Jan-16			
Day	Morning	Aftenoon	Notes	Evening
Monday				
Tuesday				
Wednesday				
Thursday				
Friday				
Saturday				
Sunday				
Week # 3	18-Jan-16 - to - 24-Jan-16			

Daily Food Diary: [Click here to enter a date.]

Breakfast	# Servings		% Daily Target	Comments
Grains				
Vegetables				
Fruits				
Dairy				
Protein				
Water				
Caffeinated Drinks				
Fruit juice				
Other...				

Lunch	# Servings		% Daily Target	Comments
Grains				
Vegetables				
Fruits				
Dairy				
Protein				
Water				
Caffeinated Drinks				
Fruit juice				
Other...				

Save Our Bones Program Weekly Progress Tracker

Dixie L Grothe

Date:	2/6/2016			2/13/2016			2/20/2016			2/27/2016		
	TRUE	Some True	Some Untrue / Untrue	TRUE	Some True	Some Untrue / Untrue	TRUE	Some True	Some Untrue / Untrue	TRUE	Some True	Some Untrue / Untrue
1. Are approximately 80% of the foods from the alkalizing column & 20% from the acidifying column.												
2. Avoided processed and refined foods and stayed away from food additives, preservatives, and artificial sweeteners.	X											
3. Avoided drinking cow's milk and other unfermented dairy products.	X											
4. Avoided drinking tap water, due to the high probability of it being fluoridated.	X											
5. Avoided drinking sodas, both diet and regular.	X											
6. Chewed my food well.												
7. Included Foundation Foods in my menu.												
8. Included some lycopene and polyphenol rich foods in my daily menu.												
9. Stopped to take a deep breath every once in a while to get extra oxygen and relieve stress.												
10. Taken all of the Foundation Supplements.												
11. Spent at least 15 minutes a day in the sun.												
12. Did aerobic weight-bearing exercises at least three times this week.												
13. Incorporated a 30 minute exercise session with light free weights twice this week.												
14. Set aside time each day for stress-reducing activities.												
15. Incorporated five behavioral changes listed in Chapter 14 *												

* Behavioral Changes listed in RELAX & HAVE FUN were:	EXAMPLE
1. Breathe	1.4.5.7.8
2. Set aside time for yourself every day	
3. Read something uplifting every morning	
4. Take a few minutes each day to be in silence with nature	
5. Remember that less is more	
6. Let go of worry and do not live with fear	
7. Laugh often	
8. Get rid of the urge to be "perfect"	
9. The only person you can change is yourself	
10. Take time to count your blessings and focus on the positive	

Chapter 7 – What can you expect? Choose life!!

I've already mentioned the importance of doing anything with a positive attitude like "this is good, this will work, the effort is worth the results, etc." It's so much more effective than having an attitude such, "this is dumb, it won't work, it takes too long, etc." Your attitude changes your body chemistry positively or negatively. One is the way of life the other is the way of death: CHOOSE LIFE!!

Choose to be positive and you'll have better success. If you're not already aware that body chemistry changes with whether you're happy, sad, or indifferent, look into it. Your body actually responds to your thoughts, positively or negatively.

Laughter is beneficial so find things you like to do that make you happy. Be lighthearted – be forgiving, be helpful, be busy, and feed your mind good things. You won't have time to think about your problems. Pretty soon, as you move ahead with the changes, you'll feel better.

And remember to track your progress. It reminds you of where you were, what you've already done, what is going right and what isn't so you can put more effort into what's working. Keep your goals in mind.

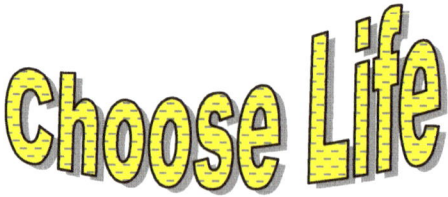

Chapter 8 – Why do you do what you do? Understand your actions...

It's important to understand "why" you are doing something so you aren't just on automatic pilot or blindly trying anything that comes along – there's a reason why certain things build up immunity and others tear it down. Ask God if this is something that would help achieve your goals.

Motivation – I wanted better health and energy for (both my husband and) me, not necessarily losing weight. Once I learned more about what's good for us and why, it became less about weight and more about feeling energized and ready to take on the day. When I finally got serious about health and nutrition and applied it, each of us lost 15 pounds in 3 months, without doing anything but changing the way we ate food. For us at the time, it was *"Fit For Life"*. Since then, I've combined different health concepts successfully based on a specific need at the time.

Boredom – The key to sticking with any health routine is variety so if you need interesting recipes, there are many suitable methods and guidelines for preparing food both on a budget and on limited time. You may find it helpful at first to refrain from introducing too many new foods to your diet until you can determine how they affect you. I discovered that when I quit eating wheat, the symptoms of IBS (irritable bowel syndrome) stopped in 1 week. Nothing else changed so I knew this was the cause of it. Evaluate how you're feeling along the way.

Establish core values – Logically evaluate what means the most to you and decide to make them work. There's that word again…DECIDE. Be serious about what you want in your life, and expect positive and lasting change. Then stick to those ideas until you achieve your goals.

Dieting – Forget about calories. The problem with dieting and counting calories is that it's not accurate unless you have the exact manufacturer, ingredients, and weights. Then when you do lose weight and quit counting calories, you end up gaining back the weight, thus the yo-yo effect. Anyway, do you really want to count calories for the rest of your life? Besides, counting calories doesn't address the real issue – good nutrition! There are better ways to lose weight and it has to do with eating right so when you start building a healthy lifestyle, the weight will come off if you're too heavy or you'll gain it if you are too thin.

Comparisons – Don't be tempted to compare your body to someone else's body. You don't have to be like models in a fashion magazine that look like they might fall over from starvation at any moment. Consider this – there are many different body types and that's the way it was designed. Imagine the boredom if everyone was the same. Be you but don't let that be an excuse for not doing anything. Find the balance.

Remember when – how many times do we recall our past? Maybe your past is pleasant, maybe not. Forget the past – it's gone now and there's nothing you can do about it either way. Move ahead and find the good in this day.

It's not yours – It's actually foreign! The immune system sends out an army of white blood cells to reject foreign matter! Disease is foreign to the body. Beware of claiming disease such as *my* osteoporosis, *my* thyroid issues, *my* heart problem, *my* gallbladder issue, *my* whatever! You're not in denial if you say you've developed a disease because your immune system needs a tune-up. Who knows? It may start a conversation that could help someone else work on their health. Maybe they don't know there are options for good health to claim and utilize.

Follow your heart – There's a misgiving going around that your heart will lead you in the right way. If the heart is always right, then why are so many people ending in divorce? Is this a logical notion – does it build a lasting relationship if you are always subject to what your "heart" tells you this moment? Emotional states fluctuate. You might be "in love" one minute and embittered the next. Make sure your heart is right before you start following it. Don't need any dry bones here…

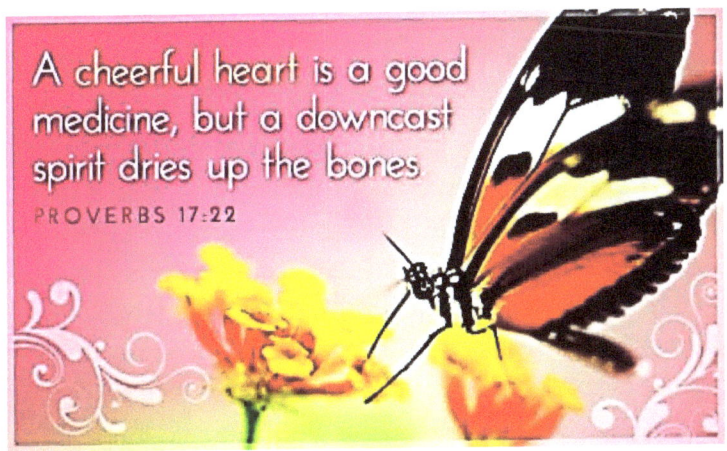

A cheerful heart is a good medicine, but a downcast spirit dries up the bones

PROVERBS 17:22

Chapter 9 – Can you shift gears? Remember, you're driving...

Sometimes things happen that change the course of action for a while. This may impact habits you've built to improve your health or maintain it. An accident, surgery, or an emotional setback of some kind, like the loss of a family member, can influence what you do for a while.

You're still in the driver's seat and need to point your car in the direction you want to go. Use the brakes and steer your life as best you can in the direction you want to go. Sometimes you need to let someone you trust help take the pressure off. If you have someone who can help in those urgent times of need, that's great, but having a backup plan is always a good idea. Professional help can save your life.

You may have heard someone say, "Plan for the worst, but expect the best". Nine times out of ten, the worst won't happen if you're prepared. Why? We do things out of fear that are counterproductive to our plans. They would turn out fine if we just left it alone. We tend to be overly concerned or exaggerate issues so preparation takes some of the stress off...it alleviates fear.

Secondly, it won't come as a shock or surprise if it does happen. Human tendency is to react emotionally at first. If you do things out of fear, it keeps you from thinking and you go into the fight or flight mode, both of which are highly stressful on your body. So take the stress out by setting up options for life's situations.

Your initial reaction will relax into logic when you remember your backup plan.

Thirdly, you can choose options in your backup plan without having to do all of them. Pause. Pray. Take a breath and think about the priorities. Do the first one, second, etc. A backup plan in case of emergency keeps us at peace because we know we've thought it through as much as possible. "We do our best and let God do the rest."

Fourthly, if you have a plan, you'll likely be ready to help others in need, too. Life can be difficult for the best of us sometimes but you can turn it around if you stay calm and find ways to help others.

Notes:

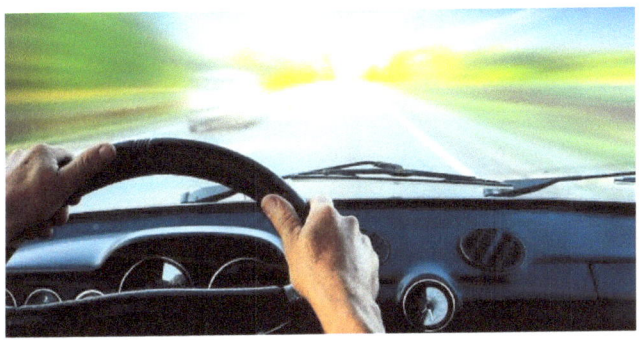

Chapter 10: Victory or defeat? Stay healthy...

Even though things in life happen that affect you physically, mentally or emotionally, you can remember the large or small steps you've made toward good health and stay healthy by keeping track of results. Sometimes people get talked out of the small or even large victories in life, giving up something they've worked so hard to achieve. Having a journal is so important in checking back on your progress.

We need to be reminded of how far we've come; what works, what doesn't, whom to consult, whom to politely ignore, see the balance, and encourages us to keep going no matter what happens. We need to remember perseverance achieves wonders when applied day after day. (That, my friends, is how I got my college degree; I'm convinced of it.)

Another important thing to remember is that if you go off your plan one day, just pick it up the next and don't get bogged down because you "fell off the wagon". Just pick up and get back on the horse.

It really doesn't take a lot of brains or even a lot of common sense to be healthy and stay there if you continue to do the things you know to do:

- Read the Bible for positive support; apply it to life

- Pray or meditate thankfully

- Be with people who support and encourage you

- Drink water as needed

- Eat the proper amount of food (balanced)

- Eat the proper proportions of greens to carbs or protein

- Do something you enjoy to get you moving

- Get fresh air and sun

- Get some sleep – 8 or 9 hours a night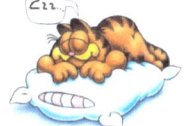

Life is 100% spiritual but a healthy body needs 80% nutrition and 20% exercise. Once you're on your way to better health, you're set up for success. Follow up on any ideas you read here, thoughts you might have had, or other things in you picked up in your research or in talking with professionals.

If you let God work in you, follow direction from professionals, diligently search out how to restore your health, and implement it regularly, you will

"Live a Lifetime of Good Health"

Actions based on goals:

1)

2)

3)

4)

5)

6)

7)

8)

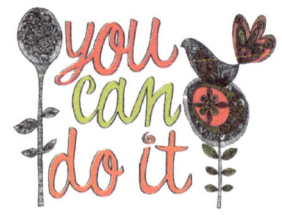